Fitness Motivation

The Ultimate Motivation Guide:

Fitness, Exercise, Motivation, and Goals

Build Lean Muscle through Discipline and Determination

By

I0425520

Nicholas Bjorn

Nicholas Bjorn

reliable, and complete information. No warranties of any kind are expressed or implied. Readers acknowledge that the author is not engaging in the rendering of legal, financial, medical, or professional advice.

Table of Contents

Introduction 7

Chapter 1: Importance of Exercising 9

So How Often Should You Exercise? 13

Chapter 2: Habits of Successful Exercisers 17

Discipline and Determination.. 22

Chapter 3: How Motivation Works 25

Phases of Motivation Needed to Get Things Done 25

Motivation Suffers When You Hate the Activities...............27

Learning About the Fear that Paralyzes You 28

Counteracting Fear.. 29

External and Internal Motivation 30

Surround Yourself with External Motivation 31

Successfully Building Internal Motivation 32

Advantages of Focusing on Your Motivation......................33

Chapter 4: How to Stay Motivated 35

Chapter 5: How to Set Fitness and Weight Loss Goals..39

Set Goals Using the S.M.A.R.T. Philosophy 39

Goals Need to be Specific and Clear *40*

Goals Need to be Measurable *40*

Goals Need to be Attainable and Realistic *41*

Goals Need to Have a Timeline *42*

Chapter 6: Creating a Fitness Plan and Staying Motivated **45**

How Do You Stay Focused When You Start to Get Bored? 46

Strategies to Keep You Going 48

Chapter 7: Introduction to How Calories Work **53**

What Calories Are 53

Breaking Down Calories in Food 54

Our Daily Caloric Needs 55

Chapter 8: Sample Exercise Routine **59**

Conclusion **63**

Introduction

I want to thank you and congratulate you for purchasing this book, "Fitness Motivation: The Ultimate Motivation Guide: Fitness, Exercise, Motivation, and Goals – Build Lean Muscle through Discipline and Determination."

This book contains proven steps and strategies on how to successfully be fitter and healthier by staying focused and motivated to reach your fitness and weight loss goals.

Anyone can achieve their fitness goals if they put their minds to it. The tasks involved in achieving your fitness goals become easier if you know how to set goals. This book will discuss how to set ideal goals, along with how motivation will improve your performance. It also discusses how the different types of motivation play a part in your success.

The methods suggested in this book are proven to keep you focused and motivated. You should start reading today to begin achieving your fitness and weight loss goals.

Thanks again for purchasing this book; I hope you enjoy it!

Nicholas Bjorn

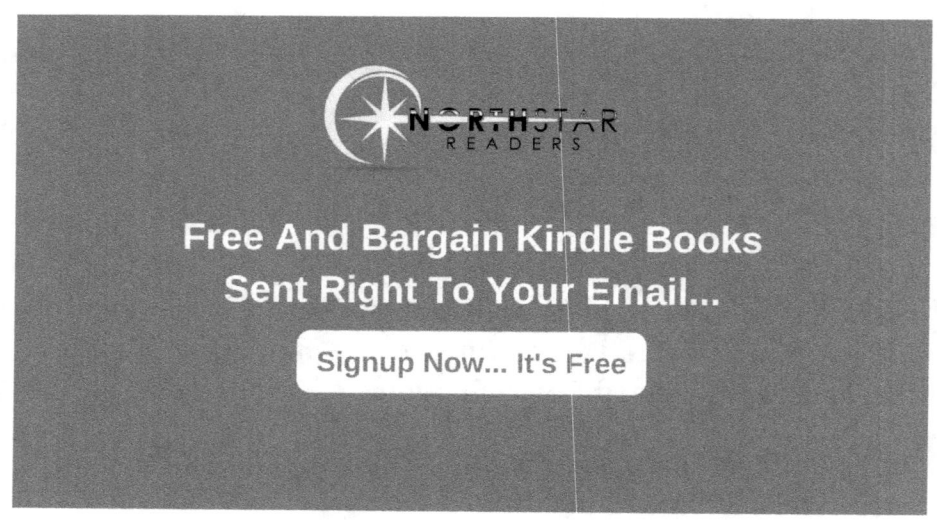

Chapter 1: Importance of Exercising

Exercise is very important. It's not enough to have a good diet alone. Diet and nutrition are the right places to start, but in order for you to have a physically fit body, you need to incorporate exercise into your lifestyle. This book is all about staying focused and motivated to reach your fitness and weight loss goals. However, before we start with the ways on how you can achieve success, let us first discuss why exercise is important aside from allowing you to lose weight.

Have you ever had a friend who seemed to never be able to gain weight? He or she always looked so slender and healthy, but his or her diet seemed very unhealthy, and he or she never exercised. Being thin is not the only measure of health. In fact, a slim person can be just as physically unfit as an obese person. The key in both cases is a lack of exercise. Aside from helping you maintain a healthy weight, exercise also promotes healthy muscle tone, joint health, and stress relief, as well as cures a variety of mood disorders.

Your body is meant to move; this is why exercising and/or playing sports is so important to your health. If you exercise on a regular basis, you will avoid developing diseases. Exercising helps reduce the risk of cancer, heart disease, diabetes, high blood pressure, and a lot of other chronic diseases. It can delay your aging process and significantly improve your appearance.

Keep in mind that staying active enables you to boost the high-density lipoprotein or good cholesterol in your body. Likewise, it helps reduce your unhealthy triglycerides. Exercising helps keep your blood flowing smoothly and decreases your risk of heart diseases. Regular physical activities actually help you prevent and manage a wide array of health issues, including depression, metabolic syndrome, stroke, and arthritis.

In addition, exercise improves your stamina. Your body uses energy to keep moving when you exercise. You can perform aerobic exercises that involve rhythmic and continuous physical motion, such as cycling and walking. Exercising boosts your stamina by training your body to use less energy and be more efficient. When your conditioning level rises, your breathing rate and heart rate go back to resting levels much sooner after doing strenuous physical activities.

You become more energized because regular physical activity can increase your endurance and muscle strength. Physical activity and exercise deliver nutrients and oxygen to your tissues, which is why your cardiovascular system is able to work more efficiently. When your lungs and heart function more efficiently, you are able to use more energy for your daily tasks.

Aside from strengthening your muscles, exercise also tones them. When you exercise using weights, as well as other forms of resistance training, you are able to develop your bones, ligaments, and muscles for greater endurance and strength. You can also improve your posture and make your muscles more toned and firm. Through exercise, you can look and feel good about yourself.

Moreover, exercise enhances your flexibility. If you want to improve your posture, you should do stretching exercises. These exercises keep your body limber, so you can twist, bend, and reach. This will reduce your chances of injury, as well as improve your coordination and balance. If you have tense and stiff body areas, such as your neck or upper back, performing stretches can help loosen up your muscles, thereby making you feel more relaxed.

Often, our aches and pains are what keep us from exercising. Once you find out that exercise can actually help alleviate those aches and pains, you will enjoy and look forward to it! Take knee joint issues, for example. A lot of knee pain and joint weakness stems from the lack of toned muscle tissue surrounding the joint. With exercise and training, you can build the muscles needed to support your joints, and you will be amazed at how much more ability, flexibility, and longevity you will have without the accompanying pain.

Exercising can help you lose weight and maintain your ideal weight. Whenever you engage in physical activity, you burn calories. Basically, the more intense your physical activity is, the more calories you burn. If you cannot work out, you should at least try to exert more effort in your normal day-to-day activities, such as walking instead of taking a cab, taking the stairs instead of the elevator, and completing more household chores or tasks.

Take note that stress can also have a negative impact on your body. In fact, studies have shown that stress can lead to a variety of chronic diseases. So if you want to live longer, you should eliminate stress as much as possible. Exercising on a regular basis can help you do just that.

Brisk walking for 30 minutes or working out at the gym can boost your mood and spirits. Have you ever noticed that before exercise, you feel down, you don't really want to exert the effort to do it, and you would rather just stay put? Then after you exercise, all of a sudden, your mood lifts, and you feel like you could take on the world? This is because exercise produces endorphins that can make you feel happier and more relaxed. The release of epinephrine, or adrenaline, is another reason for this.

Sleep is also crucial for good health. If you have trouble sleeping, regular physical activity can help. However, you should not make a habit of exercising just before you go to bed. As mentioned above, exercise can give you an adrenaline rush, which puts your body on alert and prevents you from being able to fall asleep quickly. Rather than exercising right before you go to bed, you should exercise a few hours before bedtime or after you get home from school or work. Of course, exercise first thing in the morning is also a great option and can be the perfect kick-starter for your day.

Furthermore, exercise can be a fun way to socialize and spend more time with family and friends. Exercising with a group can be much more fun than exercising alone. Besides, having someone to exercise with can motivate you toward achieving your fitness and weight loss goals. Knowing you will be missing out on a date or leaving a friend hanging if you skip your routine will help you maintain your exercising schedule. You can also exercise through sports, such as soccer and baseball, or by attending dance classes.

So How Often Should You Exercise?

Keep in mind that exercise needs to be incorporated into your lifestyle if you want to live happily and healthily. Its benefits will diminish if it is frequently disrupted. Having a stop-start routine is ineffective and can cause injuries. So if you want to achieve your desired results, you have to be consistent with your exercise.

Then again, you should also realize that exercising too often is also bad for your body. If you exercise more than you have to, you can be at risk of having tendon or muscle strains, fitness level plateaus, and loss of lean tissue. So the main question is, how often should you exercise?

To determine this, you need to look at your starting point. The exercise routine of someone who has been exercising regularly all his or her life will look quite different from that of someone who has just started a routine. However, that doesn't mean that one routine is right, and the other isn't. In each case, the person exercising must determine for himself or herself what his or her limits are.

If you used to live a sedentary lifestyle and have only just begun exercising, you need to start slowly. Do not force yourself to do strenuous physical activity if you are not ready because doing so will only lead to injuries. Three days a week for 20 minutes is recommended; this is safe, effective, and realistic. Also, make sure that you don't overdo it in those 20 minutes. It is better to start out walking a mile and getting your heart rate up to a reasonable rate than trying to run it as quickly as possible and killing yourself in the process.

You will find that over time, your stamina will improve, and you will be able to exercise at a faster pace and for a longer time and more frequently without disturbing your heart rate as much as it would have at the beginning.

On the other hand, if you are consistently active, you can complete cardio or aerobic exercises, such as cycling, jogging, or walking for up to 200 minutes a week with no more than 60 minutes per session being recommended. For example, you could choose to exercise for 40 minutes, five days a week, and take the weekend off. Others prefer to stick to only exercising three days a week, but make it an hour workout each time. Or you could keep your routine simple at a half an hour, and do it for six days a week, taking one day off.

When it comes to weight training, you should not lift weights for more than three times a week. It is not ideal to target the same muscle groups. Instead, you should aim to exercise the same muscle groups during non-consecutive days. Remember that your muscles need sufficient time to recover, and they cannot be trained effectively if they are sore or tired. For this reason, many people enjoy a schedule where they do aerobic exercises three days a week and do weight training on the two off-days in between. For example, you may go for a run on Mondays, Wednesday, and Fridays and then have a leg day on Tuesdays and an arm and ab day on Thursdays for weight training.

You should also include stretching as part of your exercise program. Stretching will improve your flexibility, which in turn increases the range of motion in your joints. These will both improve your performance and reduce the risk of injury. Each stretch should be held for at least 30 seconds and as much as 1 minute per stretch. Make sure to stretch at least all the muscles that you are planning on exercising that day. For aerobic exercise, you should ensure that you stretch all muscle groups sufficiently, as this type of exercise impacts the entire body.

In general, it is ideal to exercise at least 30 minutes each day. However, if your goal is to lose weight or meet other specific goals, you can exercise more. Do not forget to consult your doctor regarding the most suitable exercise programs for you, especially if you have not exercised for a long time or you have an existing medical condition, such as heart disease, arthritis, or diabetes.

Nicholas Bjorn

Chapter 2: Habits of Successful Exercisers

A lot of people want to exercise in the hopes of achieving their fitness and weight loss goals. However, many of them only become active in the beginning. Over time, they lose interest and motivation. If you truly want to be fitter and healthier, you need to stay motivated. The key to being able to exercise on a regular basis is to find your inner enforcer. Kelly McGonigal, PhD, a fitness instructor and health psychologist, says that getting creative and tapping your natural motivations is crucial in exercising.

If you want to achieve your exercise goals, you should not put away your fitness equipment or workout gear. You may think that putting away your gear has no impact on the way you exercise, but it actually has. When you see your fitness equipment and workout gear, your brain automatically registers exercise. Visual cues are actually a wake-up call to the brain.

The moment you see your workout clothes, sneakers, dumbbells, yoga mat, or jump rope, you become mentally ready to exercise. Hence, you should place your gear in a spot where you can easily see it, such as near your bathroom or at the foot of your bed. You can also place it in an area where you spend a lot of time during the day.

Another habit of fit people is turning their commute into a workout. Simple movements, such as running, biking, and walking can already do wonders for your health. Instead of taking a cab to your workplace, you can just walk or ride a bike. Michelle Fortier, PhD, a professor of health sciences at the University of Ottawa, agrees that turning your commute into a workout is both effective and time-efficient for people who are busy.

If your commute is so far that driving the car is the only option, you will need to find other ways to incorporate exercise into your daily life. This may mean getting up a little earlier in the morning to go for a run before leaving for work. If your job is tough, you may not have the energy at the end of a long day to motivate yourself. Remember, though, that if you do get up the motivation at the end of the day, exercise will replenish your energy.

If you have a dog, it is a great idea to exercise while you are taking it for a walk. This could mean simply going for a walk or taking your dog along for a run. This will keep both of you healthy and give your dog the outlet that it needs to burn off some energy. A well-exercised pet will always be a better behaved pet.

It is also a good idea to invest in proper workout clothes. While you can exercise in anything that feels comfortable, you should still pick clothes that offer a lot of support. For instance, you need to invest in a good sports bra or a pair of running shoes. Wearing the right kinds of clothes while working out will let you exercise better and help prevent injuries.

There is a reason why there are many different types of exercise clothes and shoes. Running shoes, for example, are built to keep up with the demands of the constant rolling motion of your feet. Shoes for playing basketball, on the other hand, will have other aspects built into them, such as a good grip for frequent stop and go and better cushioning for jumping. Make sure that the clothes you have do not hamper your flexibility. Have you ever tried to exercise in a pair of skinny jeans? If you have, you know that it is not only extremely uncomfortable, but it also greatly impairs your ability. Yoga pants are truly the most versatile clothing item in your closet when it comes to exercise.

If you have a hectic schedule and do not want to wash your gym clothes every day, then it is advisable to invest in at least one weeks' worth of clothing. Good exercise means that you will sweat. If you aren't sweating, you aren't doing it right. If you only wash once a week, let your exercise clothes air dry before you put them in your hamper. If you don't, you'll be dealing with a very smelly and mildewy hamper before too long.

According to Patricia Moreno, a mind coach and Fitness Advisory Board member, wearing clothes that show off your assets can make you feel good just by wearing them. Exercising shirtless for guys or in just a sports bra for girls can be a great motivator. Your image may either make you feel good, or it will motivate you to lose some belly fat. It may not seem like it, but in reality, this is a win-win, regardless of what your self-image is. Hopefully, exercise can help you become truly satisfied with your own body image.

Keeping track of your workout routine is also helpful. To increase the effectiveness of your workouts, you need to keep a journal. A journal can be kept to track your personal progress, or to publicize your workout plans so that people can see them. Publicizing your workout plans will make you feel more compelled to stick to your workout because you know that people are watching your progress.

Nowadays, everyone seems to have a smartphone, and while most people use them to chat, browse Facebook, or get in touch with friends, they can also be great tools for regular exercise. For one thing, you can easily set reminders for when you are scheduled to work out. Who doesn't grab their phone and look at it whenever it vibrates or dings?

Don't turn the reminder off until you have actually completed your workout. There are also many apps available that can help you monitor your heart rate, the number of calories you have burned, and where you are in relation to your exercise goals. Social networking sites can also offer additional social support. There are many different Facebook groups and online support groups that can help you meet your goals. Sometimes, a little public recognition is all the motivation it takes to get you off your seat.

You may also want to involve causes in your fitness and weight loss goals. Pledging to do exercise can help both you and your cause. For instance, for every 5 lbs. you lose, you can pledge to donate a certain amount to your chosen charity. You can also do it the other way. For every 5 lbs. you fail to lose, you need to donate money to an organization that opposes your views.

There are also many different types of charity runs and athletic events. Have people sponsor you to enter one of these events, and you can raise money for charity while at the same time sticking to your exercise goals. If your goal is to be able to run a 5K within a certain time by the time of a particular event, then that is great motivation for you to stay on track.

According to Dean Karlan, PhD, a professor of economics at Yale, antipathies and other strong feelings can have a multiplier effect. So losing just ten dollars to an enemy can make you feel like you are losing twenty or even thirty dollars, and because you want to avoid this, you tend to work harder.

As you have learned from the previous chapter, exercising can be more fun if you have friends around. However, if you do not know anyone from your gym, you should try to make friends with the people who go there regularly. Making new friends is ideal, so you will not feel alone or left out during your workout sessions. You can even meet a new workout partner. You just have to be sociable.

Of course, working out at home is just as much of an option, even though it is often viewed as harder to maintain because you don't have to go somewhere to exercise. Going out requires a certain type of commitment, and if you are going to keep up that commitment at home, it will take even more of an effort, especially if you live by yourself. If you live with family, you can make working out a family affair. This way, you will keep each other motivated, and you will be able to life a healthier life together as a group of loved ones.

Moreover, you can stage exercise contests. If you are familiar with the reality show The Biggest Loser, then you have probably seen sweaty battles on who can exercise and diet off the most weight. So if you want to push yourself further, you should probably bet money on it. If there are money and bragging rights at stake, you may feel more motivated to achieve your fitness and weight loss objectives.

However, be careful when competing so that you don't lose site of the goal, which is to be healthy. Exercising too hard can lead to injury and health problems, and you don't want to go down that road. If you enter a competition, make sure that the guidelines and goals are reasonable. Try to take part in something that you know the other competitors are on the same level as you and that you won't be competing against an all-star athlete.

Discipline and Determination

If we look at all the habits that mark a successful exercise routine, you will quickly realize that it takes a lot of discipline and determination. No matter what type of routine you chose, you will not be able to make it without these two qualities. So how can you foster these two qualities? The answer may surprise you, as you most likely already have both of these qualities. You may just be using them on the wrong thing.

Try to think of something in your life that you succeeded at. Something that you just did not give up on until it was completed. Chances are, you can come up with something, and I can guarantee you that you did this with the help of discipline and determination.

Take reading a book, for example. Many people struggle with reading books, while others can't get enough. If you are a bookworm, then you know that reading through a massive book like Tolstoy's *War and Peace* takes an incredible amount of discipline and determination, but you wade through the heavy ideas and deep storyline and come out on the other end feeling accomplished. Your discipline and determination drove you because you were doing something that you loved. You were motivated.

This leads us to our next chapter, which is about motivation. You see, as long as you are motivated, you will never lack the discipline or the determination to complete a task. So instead of trying to reach inside yourself for some willpower that you just can't seem to muster, try taking a closer look at your motivating factors. Chances are that if you have not been able to complete a successful exercise or diet routine in the past, it was because of a lack of motivation and not a lack of ability on your part.

Nicholas Bjorn

Chapter 3: How Motivation Works

Finding a source for your motivation is essential if you want to get things done. The most difficult things in life require a lot of motivation to accomplish. With an ever increasing amount of distractions and opportunities to procrastinate around us, it is difficult to keep ourselves motivated these days.

The challenge of motivation is most evident in matters concerning our health. Given that most of the health-related tasks that need to be done have no immediately observable effects, we easily lose motivation with them. In working out, for instance, many people lose interest when they can't see any visible results after a few sessions. This leads some impatient people to look for shortcuts. Some of the weight loss shortcuts found in the market, however, have dangerous effects on our health. To avoid these types of workout methods and to keep yourself motivated, you must understand how motivation works.

Phases of Motivation Needed to Get Things Done

There are three major parts of workout tasks where motivation is essential: before starting, in the middle of the task, and before ending the task.

It usually takes a lot of motivation to start a health-related task. The amount of motivation that we need is greater if we hate the activity. This is the type of motivation needed when you are trying to convince yourself to get out of bed in the morning to start running.

Many factors affect our ability to start tasks. You may not be confident with your skills to accomplish it, and you may be planning to learn more before jumping in. It could also be because of underlying fears that cause you to procrastinate. It is also a simple scientific fact that starting any process takes the most energy – turning a light bulb on burns more energy than having a light bulb that is already on for the same amount of time. Once you get going, things will get easier, but you need to muster the energy to get started first.

However, this isn't the only time you will need energy. A lot of motivation is also needed when you are in the middle of the task. You need the motivation to keep your focus on your goal until you have accomplished it. This challenge is most difficult when the task requires a lot of time before it is done. You will need a lot of patience to keep yourself focused on the task at hand and to prevent your skeptical mind from sabotaging your success.

Working out is most definitely an exercise in patience, and it is helpful if you are able to practice patience in other areas of your life as well. If you are comfortable with being patient, then persevering over time with your exercise routine will come to you more easily.

The last phase of motivation is usually needed for the final push to get a task done. This phase of motivation prevents you from taking too many breaks when you are almost at the finish line. Have you ever noticed that long-distance athletes will often push themselves to their limit on the last lap? With the goal almost in reach, they start sprinting instead of jogging, and this takes an incredible amount of energy and willpower to accomplish. Naturally, people are vulnerable to procrastination when they are already near the end of their goals because they think that only a small amount of work is needed to get the task done. This is why giving that extra push at the end when you have almost reached your goal is especially important.

For tasks related to your fitness goals or losing weight, you will need these three phases of motivation. You need a lot of motivation to get off the couch and work out every day. You will also need the motivation to limit your calorie intake and avoid high-calorie food types. When you are already in the middle of a workout and diet program, it takes a lot of motivation for you to keep pushing to get better.

Motivation Suffers When You Hate the Activities

After working out and dieting for a while, beginners tend to start to have a negative attitude toward these tasks. They tend to hate the pain and the sweat, and this leads them to procrastinate on their scheduled workouts and fail on their meal plans when they are confronted with delicious types of food. They tend to hate waking up for a morning run or getting ready to go to the gym.

We cite a lot of reasons why we hate tasks related to losing weight, but you'll be surprised by how far off these reasons are from the primary reason. The most basic source of all our hatred toward these tasks is fear. Your mind can become a victim of modern types of fear. These fears are the biggest factors that demotivate us even before we start.

In losing weight, one of the most common challenges is the fear of failing. If you have tried losing weight in the past, and you failed at some point, you already have the thoughts of failure ingrained in your mind. When you try to do the same task in the future, this lingering fear will still remain in your mind. It will come out and do damage on your motivation when you are most vulnerable.

For most people, this is when they are in their beds, and they feel that they deserve to be resting. This is the time when we usually ask ourselves; "What's the point?" You begin to question your whole motive for working out.

Given the strong effects of fear on us during this weak mental state, we need to learn how to control our own motivation. You need to be constantly aware of your level of motivation. As long as you do this, you will have the strength to carry on in your weight loss journey.

Learning About the Fear that Paralyzes You

Motivation is not just about pushing through against laziness. It is also about dealing with the fears that you already have in your mind. Every time you are about to skip on a scheduled workout session or every time you place too much food on your plate, you should ask yourself these questions: Why am I doing this? What am I afraid of?

In the process of answering these questions, you will be able to reflect on your present attitude, and this will lead you to keep working on your goal. By analyzing your thought process, you will not only help yourself prolong your motivation but also build a state of mind that allows you to control it.

As Zig Ziglar said, motivation is not permanent. Even if you succeeded in boosting your motivation today, you will need to do it again tomorrow. That is the nature of motivation. You have to constantly work on it. You can do this by using both internal and external sources of motivation.

Counteracting Fear

It isn't enough to simply know what you are afraid of. Thousands of people live every day of their lives in fear, knowing exactly why, but few people actually work to counteract fear. In dealing with fear, the biggest weapon you have is love. Think of some things that you absolutely love. Would you go to any length to keep those things in your life? Absolutely! No matter what comes your way, love can keep you on track, and this doesn't just mean romantic love. It can also mean loving a certain hobby or activity.

For example, perhaps you love to travel. There is nothing in this life that entices you more. However, your weight and physical ailments are starting to hinder you from being able to follow that dream. In this way, your love of travel can be a profound motivator, strong enough to overcome any fear that you may have.

Of course, familial or romantic love can be incredibly motivating as well. Perhaps your health is to the point that you don't think you can go on like this and that you are of no help to your family and loved ones. However, you love them, and you want to be there for them for many years to come. This can also be an incredibly strong motivating factor in deciding to become healthy. Every time you struggle to get started, just think of the people you love, and it will seem all the more worthwhile.

External and Internal Motivation

All this process of self-reflection will help you develop strategies that will help increase your external and internal motivation. External motivation is the type of motivation that we derive from sources outside of our minds. This is the type of motivation that you experience when you feel like working out because you hear one of your favorite workout songs. The people and the things that surround us affect our external motivation. Although this type of motivation is easy to create, it doesn't last very long. We should use it together with internal motivation.

Internal motivation happens when the principles and the values that you abide to become the reasons behind your actions. If you have this type of motivation, you do not need to hear any type of music just to start working out. Though this type of motivation is more difficult to develop, you should still work on it because its effects last longer. To have a strong source of internal motivation, you need a combination of two things: constant motivation practice and a set of positive principles to follow.

Surround Yourself with External Motivation

At the beginning of your fitness or weight loss program, it is understandable that your internal source of motivation may not be strong yet. For the early part, you will need to make sure that the people and the things around you motivate you to work harder. You should also decrease the factors that demotivate you in your surroundings.

As we already mentioned, setting an alarm on your phone or mobile device is a great place to start for external motivation. Once that becomes the norm, though, you may easily just dismiss it. So work on other external factors as well. Always keep your workout clothes ready to go. Put the shoes you wear for exercising where you can see them, in a convenient location. Start getting pumped with music even before you are planning on exercising.

Perhaps you were in shape at one point, and you have a photo of what you want your body to get back to. Post that photo where you can see it as a reminder that your goals are achievable. If this is the first time in your life you are trying to become healthy, then maybe you can keep a picture of a role model around to help motivate you.

Another external motivating factor for frugal people can be money. If you spend monthly to have a gym membership but are generally tight for money or just like to watch your budget closely, then you are more likely to try and get your money's worth. Why pay for something if you're not going to use it?

Successfully Building Internal Motivation

If we're honest, probably all of us have lofty goals and standards that we try to live by. Regardless of your religion or culture, there are certain values that most humans try to attain. At the core of most of these values is living in such a way that you are making the world a better place, in one way or another. How can you use this most basic trait to build internal motivation to want to work out?

First, you will need to realize that you will never be able to live to your fullest potential without being healthy. One of the most basic things that keep us from realizing our dreams or making a difference is our health. Obesity and poor diet and exercise routines are at the root of many different health issues, as we already discussed. If you don't live a healthy life, you won't be able to make as big of an impact on the world as you otherwise would.

So how do you build internal motivation? One of the best ways of doing this is mediation. Meditation allows your mind to focus and contemplate. If you need some quiet time to reflect before your exercise routine, by all means, do so. Visualize what you can achieve and how much better your life will be if your body is functioning at its highest capacity. Use a meditation journal to jot down inspirational thoughts and ideas that you can look back on and reflect.

Another great way to foster internal motivation is by posting motivational quotes around you. If you are religious, look for quotes in your Scriptures that will help encourage you in your journey. This will help keep your mind focused on the values that you cherish. An often used text for Christians is found in 1. Corinthians 6:19-20, where it says: "Do you not know that your body is a temple of the Holy Spirit within you, whom you have from God, and that you are not your own? For you have been purchased at a price. Therefore, glorify God in your body."

If you are not religious, you may also find quotes from role models in your life to be very inspiring. There may also be some sayings that will help foster internal motivation. A few great examples would be "Fitness is not about being better than someone else, but being better than you used to be," or "You don't have to be great to start, but you have to start to be great." If you surround yourself with these types of positive ideas, then you are much more likely to maintain internal motivation.

Advantages of Focusing on Your Motivation

By learning how to focus and improve your motivation, you will learn a lot about yourself and how your mind works. You will not only learn about your fears but also where they come from and their particular effects on your behavior.

Motivation is a game changer. If you have tried and failed at starting a fitness program or losing weight in the past, learning about your motivation and practicing the principles offered in this book will significantly improve your chances.

By being aware of how motivation works, you will also develop a no-excuse mindset. Knowing that you can control your motivation prevents you from placing too much weight on uncontrollable factors in reaching your goals. You will hold yourself accountable for all your failures, and you have only yourself to thank for because of all the successes that you gain.

Chapter 4: How to Stay Motivated

If you have just made some changes in your lifestyle, then that is great news. Congratulate yourself on the effort, and do your best to stay on track. Starting an exercise routine is easy, but staying motivated can be quite difficult. So how can you stay motivated?

Well, it's important for you to determine what your motivation and goals are. You have to be clear about these. Make sure that you know exactly why you are making changes in your lifestyle. Likewise, you need to have a clear understanding of what you wish to accomplish in the end.

Keep in mind that exercising to look good should not be your only goal. Looking good, in the end, is not really enough to keep you going. If you focus on this alone, you will eventually cave in to your weakness sooner or later. If you are trying to diet, you might just give in to unhealthy food choices. After all, if you look great, but your body and health leave you feeling miserable all the time, your looks will be worth nothing. It is also important to note that different people will look differently when they are healthy. We come in all shapes and sizes, and this would still be true if everyone in the world were in perfect health.

You have to be specific on what goals you are trying to aim for. Once you figure this out, you should create a plan on how you can get there. For instance, if you want to improve your diet to improve your health, then start planning your meals.

If you want to improve your insulin sensitivity, then you need to monitor your glucose levels. If you want to lose weight and improve your appearance, then take your measurements, as well as photos of yourself, before your diet and exercise plans. The more measurable and specific your goals are, the easier it will be for you to track your progress.

One thing to look out for, though, is setting unrealistic goals. If this is the first time you are seriously looking into an exercise and diet routine, you won't know exactly what goal to set for yourself in terms of weight. You know you want to become healthy, but you're not sure at what weight you will feel satisfied with your body and healthy enough to start maintaining your weight. In this case, set smaller goals, and then go from there. For example, your first goals could be losing 20 lbs. Once you reach that goal and decide you need to lose more, set another goal for another 20 lbs., and so forth. Achieving your smaller goals can also be very fulfilling and a great motivating factor.

It is also ideal to have checkpoints. Instead of inspecting your size daily or weighing yourself weekly, you should have checkpoints every eight weeks or so. This is so you will not get hung up on the small details of your progress, and you will have a sense of internal competitiveness. You will also have sufficient time to see the results.

How can you have checkpoints? Well, if you are trying to increase your strength, lose weight, or improve your physical appearance, you can weigh yourself and test your ability in several basic exercises, such as push-ups, pull-ups, squats, and sprints. If you are trying to improve your insulin sensitivity, your checkpoints can be your fasting glucose levels.

If you are trying to improve your skin condition and get rid of eczema or allergies, your checkpoints can be the frequency of your symptoms. Checkpoints are also beneficial in a way that they let you acknowledge the fact that long-lasting health changes take time and keep you from getting discouraged when you are not active.

Another way that you could stay motivated is to be educated. It is generally helpful to remind yourself why you have a goal in the first place. Hence, you should continue to educate yourself regarding health, fitness, and nutrition. You can even ask a friend or your partner to help you stay on track by also making changes in their lives and getting educated.

Do not forget to set short-term goals as well. If you cannot jump into a new fitness or diet plan immediately, then try to set some small goals. Make sure to write these on paper so you will not forget. Whenever you achieve a goal, start on another one right away. You can reward yourself by buying something new or going to a spa. Reaping rewards for achieving short-term goals can keep you motivated in achieving your long-term goal.

You should also make exercising a habit. Healthy living is actually easier if you make it part of your regular routine. Once you form a habit, exercising and dieting will no longer feel like obligations. You will be used to doing them, and your body will automatically act. Moreover, you will not think of an end point each time you reach a goal. Instead, your mind will be centered on your lifestyle change. You will find that after a while, exercising will come naturally as part of your day, just like brushing your teeth or showering. Once that is the case, it will be a lot harder for you to quit, and motivation will not be nearly as essential as it was at the beginning of your journey.

Another thing to remember when keeping motivated is that you don't want to have a single event in your life as your only goal or motivating factor. For example, many people set it as a goal to lose a certain amount of weight to look perfect on their wedding day, but once that goal is reached, they fall back into their old ways and quickly gain back the pounds they lost. To avoid this, make sure that your fitness goals aren't entirely built around one event. You need to incorporate your goals into your lifestyle to be successful.

Chapter 5: How to Set Fitness and Weight Loss Goals

Goals and life organization are important in every area of life. The most successful people will tell you that they didn't get where they are today by just spontaneously doing life. Without goals, you have nothing concrete to shoot for, and you will just be blowing in the wind.

Well-planned fitness and weight loss goals can help you transform your thoughts into action. Such goals can actually mean the difference between failure and success. Well-planned goals that are specific, measurable, and realistic will keep you motivated and focused. They will also give you a plan for change as you develop a healthier lifestyle. On the other hand, overly aggressive and unrealistic weight loss goals will just undermine your efforts.

Set Goals Using the S.M.A.R.T. Philosophy

So how can you set ideal fitness and weight loss goals? First of all, you need to set *smart* goals. The S.M.A.R.T. philosophy is an ideal tool to use to set goals. The S.M.A.R.T. acronym stands for:

- **S**pecific

- **M**easurable

- **A**ttainable

- **R**ealistic

- **T**imeline

Goals Need to be Specific and Clear

Write down all your thoughts, and include specific details. When do you plan to start, and where do you want to do it? How will you fit your workout into your hectic schedule? What are the things that you need to get started? You can use these questions as guidelines in planning your fitness and weight loss goals.

You can't just set your goal as: "I want to lose weight." That won't work. Your goal needs to be specific about HOW MUCH weight or HOW MANY inches you want to lose. If you aren't sure of your end goal, set a goal that you know is within your reach. Once you reach that goal, you can move on to the next one.

Goals Need to be Measurable

Measurable goals are ones that you can use to track your progress. How far do you plan to walk, and for how long? How much time do you plan to devote to your exercise session? How many days a week will you spend walking? How many pounds do you want to lose? What size clothes do you want to fit into? You can't manage your goals if you don't measure them. You also have to review your progress each week so you can determine how far you have come. By having a specific weight loss goal, you can manage that goal and change the plan if necessary.

To measure accurately, you will need to keep some sort of journal or record, and you will also want to be in possession of an accurate scale. Doing this and seeing results will also continue to motivate you to move forward with your workout plan. Once again, simply saying "I want to lose weight," or, "I want to feel healthy," shouldn't be the extent of your goal.

Goals Need to be Attainable and Realistic

It is also important to focus on what is relevant and attainable to you. Your goals should be within your capabilities. If you set unrealistic goals, you're setting yourself up for failure. See to it that you also consider your limitations, health concerns, fitness level, and available time, among other vital factors. You will be able to come up with achievable goals if you tailor your expectations to your situation. Create goals that give you confidence in achieving them, rather than setting goals that you doubt are possible to reach.

For most people, an attainable goal is losing 5% to 10% of their current weight or 1 to 2 lbs. per week. However, if that isn't you, don't beat yourself up about it. First, lower your expectations, and then you will be able to more clearly see the progress you are making. It is better to set numerous small goals that help motivate you than to set one large goal that seems impossible to achieve and depresses you every time you think about it.

Goals Need to Have a Timeline

Of course, timing is also very important. Timing can make the difference between failure and success. Choose a specific start date for your plans, and try hard not to keep putting that date off. This date is your deadline by which you need to achieve your goal. It should create pressure and a sense of urgency to keep you focused and motivated. Make sure that you also account for circumstances that may hamper your efforts, such as school or work demands, relationship problems, and vacations. In order to avoid hassles, you may want to resolve all issues before starting.

You need these time deadlines to keep you moving forward. Setting timelines and goals that are too easy to achieve is also a common pitfall, as they won't cause you to stretch your ability. You want to become a fitter, healthier, and better person than you were before, and you won't be able to achieve that without some effort. If you aren't breaking a sweat, you're doing something wrong.

You should focus more on the process instead of the outcome. Make the most out of your exercise routines, and quit thinking of how you will feel or look like in the end. Keep in mind that changing your process, habits, and behaviors are crucial for reaching your fitness and weight loss goals. The key to achieving your goals are not necessarily focusing on your target results or weight.

It is also helpful to anticipate setbacks. Remember that setbacks are a natural part of behavior change and life in general. People who have successfully made changes in their lives have experienced setbacks at some point. To help you stay or return on course, identify and overcome potential setbacks as soon as they occur.

You also have to adjust and reassess your goals whenever necessary. Be willing to change them as you achieve progress, and adjust your goals to fit your new fitter and healthier lifestyle.

Nicholas Bjorn

Chapter 6: Creating a Fitness Plan and Staying Motivated

Creating a fitness plan can encourage you to stick to your fitness and weight loss goals. It is easy to plan and dream of achieving success. However, it is very difficult to start and stick to a fitness plan. You have learned from the previous chapters how you can create an ideal fitness plan and how you can stay motivated in exercising, but how can you stay motivated with your fitness plan, and how can you get back on track when you start to lose motivation?

Well, you can start with wearing snug and stylish workout clothes. It is very important for your clothes to fit properly and provide support. Nonetheless, it would not hurt to wear fashionable workout clothes to make you look good and feel great about yourself. To cushion your feet, make sure that you wear comfortable socks and shoes. Choose your shoes according to your type of workout. For instance, you can choose running shoes, aerobic shoes, cross trainers, etc.

If the weather is cold, you can wear layers of clothing to keep you warm. If it is hot and humid outside, you can wear gym clothes made of cotton to keep you cool. You may also want to ask other people to exercise with you. People tend to stick to their workout routines better when they have a workout partner. When you know that someone else is counting on you, you tend to commit and not slack off during sessions.

How Do You Stay Focused When You Start to Get Bored?

Unfortunately, not all people who start a weight loss journey get to the end. Most of them lose interest halfway through the program. They just no longer feel motivated enough, which is why they go back to their old ways. These people cannot seem to maintain consistency for a long period of time. They also tend to struggle with mental endurance, which is why they are having a hard time following through.

Athletes may be physically fit because of their genetics. However, genetics are not everything. These athletes also become successful in achieving their fitness goals because they can efficiently deal with the boredom of daily training. Doing the same lifts over and over can certainly test your patience.

To stay motivated with your workout, you need to have unstoppable willpower and passion. There is no magic pill for staying inspired and motivated every day. You just have to prevent your emotions from determining your actions. Successful exercisers always find a way to show up and work through the boredom. They are able to exercise every day, no matter what happens.

Your ability to do work when it is not easy is what separates you from everyone else. It is practically the difference between amateurs and professionals. So if you want to level yourself with professional athletes and successful exercisers, you should do your best to beat boredom and work your way towards your fitness goals. Do not give up when you feel like doing so.

Moreover, remind yourself that it is the process and not the event that is important. All too often, people think that their goals are only about results. They view success as an event that can be completed and achieved. For instance, some people view health as an event. They think that if they lose 20 lbs., they will be in shape. Well, this is not really true.

If you want to achieve goals consistently, you have to realize that it is not the results or the events that make the difference. Instead, it is your commitment to the process that counts. Focus on your daily workout and not the single event. You should be connected deeply with exercising that doing it does not make you feel uncomfortable or uninspired. You have to love exercising.

Media is a great way to keep your mind active during workouts and make them seem less boring. Whether it be listening to workout music or an audio book, or catching up on your latest show, you can use media to pass the time on a long run that you have already done 100 times and has become boring.

Another way to keep things interesting is to compete against yourself. At each workout, see if you can outperform your last workout. Maybe you will run the mile just one second faster, or perhaps you will do just one more push-up. Whatever it is, keeping track of your stats and competing against yourself can always keep it interesting. Of course, if you are working out with someone else, you can also keep the competition going there, and having someone for conversation is never a bad idea to get through the boredom.

Strategies to Keep You Going

In order for you to be able to stick to a workout routine, you need to have a reason to carry on when you feel like quitting. So how can you keep going when you no longer think you can finish your session? Here are some simple strategies that you can do.

You can recharge your exercise motivation. You should not allow any mental hurdles to stand between you and what you want to achieve. If you want to lose weight, then do not let anyone or anything get in the way of your success. If you ever encounter setbacks, try your best to overcome them. Make sure that you steer around slim-down excuses and speed bumps.

You have to reboot your motivation to exercise. If you encounter small problems, you may use them as an excuse to just quit. For instance, if your weighing scale gets stuck, you may take that as a sign to stop. Well, if you have this kind of mentality, you will not get far in your fitness and weight loss journey. You have to change your mindset regarding these things.

Moreover, you should always think that you can do it. You can lose excess weight. According to a study at the University of Minnesota, people who watch their waistlines and weigh themselves more often are able to lose weight faster than those who do not. While it may not be ideal to watch your progress daily, you should try to weigh yourself every week to notice how far you have come in your journey.

See to it that you also rev up your routine. Remember that as your metabolism shifts to accommodate your smaller size, you need to change what you do in order to coax your body to keep shedding fat. If you are already eating lightly, you should not cut back more. Instead, you should turn up the intensity of your workout sessions or make your exercise time longer. Keep stretching yourself and your ability. You may be surprised out how amazing your core strength and stamina may become.

Whenever you work out, you should always psych yourself up. This is especially true with strength training. According to a study at the School of Sport and Exercise Science at the Wintec, Waikato Institute of Technology, you can increase your muscle power by 8% if you psych yourself up when you do strength training. If you visualize yourself having perfect lifts, you will be able to reap about 12% more power.

Then again, if you cannot do more repetitions at the same weight, you can go lighter. Simply reduce the amount that you lift in 10% increments until you finish your set with good form. Keep in mind that form is crucial. If your form is poor, you can be at risk of injury.

When running or jogging for distance, it is alright to slow down. However, it is not alright to stop. Slow down but keep going. You can recite a mantra in your mind to help you focus better on your workout. Tell yourself that you are a running machine and that you can run as far as you can.

Alternatively, running or jogging in intervals is ideal to improve performance. Split your run into two parts: running and walking. You can jog one quarter of a mile and then walk for half a mile before finishing off by jogging another quarter. As you improve, you should stretch out your jogging and reduce your walking segment before finishing the final quarter mile. You can do this three to four times a week. You will be surprised at how good you will become after just six weeks. Within that timeframe, you will be able to run the entire distance.

Always try to stay in rhythm. Breathing properly is very important and can be just as powerful as a mantra. Match your inhales and exhales to the number of strides you are taking. For example, take four steps as you inhale, and then another four as you exhale. As you get more tired, your breathing will speed up, but keep it in rhythm. By the end, you may be inhaling every two steps instead of four.

Breathing steadily can also increase concentration and awareness of your body, which can help prevent injury and side stitches. If you do end up with a side stitch while exercising, don't stop completely and sit down. Rather, fold your hands behind your head and keep on walking or running at a slow pace.

Correct posture is also extremely important when working out and will keep your body in better shape, allowing you to continue with your exercise regimen as planned. Each type of exercise will have a different form or posture that is correct. Of course, the most common posture we think of is our posture when standing. Your feet should be facing forward, with your legs extending straight down from your hips. To find your center, stretch out your arms above your head until you can clasp your hands. Your arms will naturally position themselves straight up. Unclasp your hands and bring your arms down on either side while keeping them extended until they are horizontal with the floor. Then let your arms fall to your sides. The position you are in now is a correct posture.

Moreover, you should not get discouraged when you hurt your body. Some people hurt their knees, and they end up stopping for a month. If you stop exercising for just three days, your body already starts to lose its conditioning abilities. All your initial efforts will just be wasted if you stop halfway. If you do not feel motivated enough to keep going, remind yourself that there is more than one way to achieve your goal.

Dr. Trent Petrie, director of the Center for Sports Psychology at the University of North Texas, suggests that you write down all your negative thoughts, and reframe them into positive ones. For instance, if you can't run due to a sore ankle, you can write that down and then reframe it by wanting to go cycling or doing a spin class instead.

Your injury should not stop you from working out because there are plenty of alternatives you can try. Then again, if simply bending your knee causes great pain, you should consult your doctor.

Nicholas Bjorn

Chapter 7: Introduction to How Calories Work

Aside from exercising, maintaining a balanced diet is also important if you want to achieve your fitness and weight loss goals. What you eat will have a significant impact on how you look and perform.

Any effective weight loss diet follows this simple rule: eat less, and burn more calories. What you do eat needs to be packed with healthy nutrients and minerals. Cutting back on what you eat and still just eating junk food is not going to do much to improve your health. You want to be able to gain the most nutrition from the least number of calories possible. So what is a calorie? Understanding this will show you the crucial role that nutrition plays in losing weight and gaining lean muscle.

What Calories Are

The dictionary definition of a "calorie" is this: it is a unit or quantity of heat that is needed to raise the temperature of 1 gram of water by 1 degree Celsius (or 1.8 degrees Fahrenheit) at atmospheric pressure.

The "calories" used in food are actually kilo-calories, and 1 kilo-calorie is equal to 1,000 calories. This means if a box of cookies has 140 calories per serving; it actually means 140,000 actual calories. Nutritionists use the word "calories" to describe the energy-producing potential in food, and it is these calories that fuel all of our bodily functions.

The "calories" in exercise also mean the same: if a fitness chart states that you will burn 100 calories for each mile that you run, it actually means you burn 100,000 calories or 100 kilo-calories. Hence, when the word "calorie" is mentioned in this book, it refers to kilo-calories.

Breaking Down Calories in Food

The number of calories in your food shows the amount of energy that you will get from it. All foods are a combination of three building blocks, namely, carbohydrates, protein, and fat, which are referred to as macro-nutrients. The calories per gram of each macro-nutrient are as follows:

- **Carbohydrates** - 4 calories

- **Protein** - 4 calories

- **Fat** - 9 calories

As fat has more than twice the number of calories present in carbohydrates and protein, it obviously means fat is more difficult to burn off; therefore, it should be consumed sparingly.

Let's take a look at the nutritional label on a box of cookies, which shows that the serving size is 25 grams, and the number of calories per serving is 120. If we open up the packet and burn up the cookies directly in an open fire and let it burn off entirely, this will produce 120 kilo-calories, enough to increase the temperature of 120 kilograms of water to 1 degree Celsius.

A closer look at the nutritional label will show you that there are 5 grams of fat, 16 grams of carbohydrates, and 3 grams of protein, which gives you a total of 24 grams (food companies tend to round off the number). Therefore, the 120 calories on the nutrition label of the cookies actually contain 45 calories from fat (5 grams multiplied by 9 calories), 64 calories from carbohydrates, and 12 calories from protein.

In order for the body to burn these 120 calories, it has to break down the carbohydrates into sugars, such as glucose, the proteins into amino acids, and the fats into fatty acids and glycerol. After this, these organic compounds are transferred via the bloodstream to the different cells in the body for immediate use, and the excess is stored for future use in the form of body fat.

Our Daily Caloric Needs

When nutritional labels show the percentages of the daily values that the body needs, they typically refer to someone who follows a 2,000-calorie diet. It is difficult to identify exactly how many calories our cells require to function properly, as each person's daily physical activities vary, along with his or her height, weight, age and, gender.

To know approximately how many calories you need to consume per day so that you can achieve your weight loss goals, there are three important factors that you need to be aware of:

1. **Basal Metabolic Rate or BMR**

As the name implies, the BMR provides you with a baseline that gives you a starting point for how many calories your body requires. It is calculated by measuring the amount of energy your body expends while at rest and while not actively digesting anything. Thus, figuring out your BMR requires a fast of at least 12 hours, so first thing in the morning isn't a bad time to figure it out. It is difficult to find out your BMR at home, but some fitness centers and doctors will offer the service. As body temperature is an important factor in the test, it is important that the test takes place in a temperature-controlled atmosphere at a comfortable temperature. The formula for calculation is quite complicated and requires the input of your gender, height, weight, and age. Once you figure out this basic number, you know the amount of energy your body needs to stay alive without any physical exertion.

2. **Physical Activity**

After having figured out your baseline, you will need to figure out how many calories your daily physical activities require. Different activities will burn different amounts of calories, and the number you come up with will be the best estimate, as an exact calculation is not possible. One thing you can do to help track your daily physical activity is to wear a step calculator that also keeps track of your heart rate. This will give you a good place to start.

3. **Thermic Effect of Food**

The thermic effect of food is the amount of energy it takes to process the food you ingest and convert it into energy for the body. Just like a motor needs fuel to bring you from point A to point B, your body needs to burn calories to fuel all its activities. You can find many different tables online that will show you the exact thermic effect of different foods.

After these three factors are calculated, they need to be added up, and then the result would be the total number of calories that your body requires each day. There are many calorie counters available online, all of which give different results based on the formulas they used. Adding the above three factors is the most accurate way of determining how many calories your body requires each day.

Once you have figured out how many calories your body requires to maintain your current status, you will want to set your daily caloric intake a little lower if you wish to lose weight. The body will only burn its fat reserves if it is not getting enough energy from what you are ingesting for your daily need. Try cutting out a couple hundred calories for starters to see what that does for your body. Give it about a month before you decide whether you want to cut more for faster weight loss or cut a little less because you are losing too much weight.

Keep in mind that as you build stamina through your exercise routine, you will burn more and more calories every day. Eventually, you may get to a point where you actually need to increase your caloric intake because you are burning enough through exercise to make up for it. This is why you often see athletes like weightlifters and football players have a daily caloric intake that is higher than that of the average person. If they did not increase the number of calories they consume, they would not have sufficient fuel for the training they are undertaking, and they would not be able to exercise as fully as they want to. Chances are, though, that it will be a while before you reach that point.

The types of calories you consume are also important. For building muscle and reducing fat deposits, you will want to increase the amount of protein and healthy fats you consume while reducing the amount of carbohydrates and sugar in your diet. Great foods for physical fitness and muscle tone include eggs rich in Omega-3 fatty acids, nuts, avocado, lean meats and fish, full-fat dairy products, and various seeds and green vegetables. Fruits are generally rich in sugar, so it is best to only enjoy them in moderation. They do make a great healthy dessert, as they are packed with important vitamins and minerals.

Chapter 8: Sample Exercise Routine

This sample is by no means a strict rulebook that you should follow. Instead, use it as a starting point for your new fit and lean lifestyle. The example given assumes that the person starting is someone who is currently active but has had no exercise routine in the past. You will notice that time is needed at the beginning toward building up stamina.

Month 1

Start out with 20-minute aerobic exercises on Monday, Wednesday, and Friday and 20-minute weight training exercises on Tuesday and Thursday. By the end of the month, you will notice your stamina increasing.

Monday – Go for a 20-minute run or walk. Remember, try to stay active the entire time; in other words, if you are tired of running, simply walk for a while, but don't stand still. You want to keep your heart rate up the entire time.

Tuesday – Leg day: Do some leg exercises, such as leg lifts, seated leg curls, leg extensions, or a seated calf raise. Start with three sets of four or five different exercises, with enough repetitions to fill your 20 minutes. The first month is all about figuring out where your body is at. By the end of the month, you will know better what you are currently capable of.

Wednesday – Do 20 minutes of Zumba, or go swimming or biking. Remember to stay active for the entire 20 minutes.

Thursday – Arm and ab day: Try curls, push-ups, pull-ups, or other simple exercises to start with. Just as with leg day, figure out how many sets and reps you are able to go through to fill your 20 minutes.

Friday – Go for another 20-minute run or walk.

At the end of the first week, you may feel like you never want to do that again. Trust me, the hardest part is now behind you. It will only get easier from here on out.

Month 2

Follow the same basic routine as outlined in month 1, but increase the duration of your workout sessions to 25 minutes each.

Month 3

Follow the same basic routine as outlined in month 1, but increase the duration of your workout sessions to 30 minutes each.

Month 4

At this point, keep going with your 30-minute routines, but try to build more challenging exercises into your weight-lifting days, and push yourself to best your time when running on your aerobic days. You should be able to see an improvement every week.

I hope this gives you a good idea of where to start. The pace at which you will progress will vary for everyone individually. Find what is right for you, and you will actually start enjoying your daily workout routine. It will become part of who you are, and your body will feel better than it ever has before.

Nicholas Bjorn

Conclusion

Thank you again for purchasing this book!

I hope this book was able to help you achieve your fitness and weight loss goals by providing you with ways to stay focused and motivated.

The next step is to apply what you have learned from this book. There is no better time than now to get started on a healthier and more active lifestyle. Create a fitness plan, and set goals using the S.M.A.R.T. philosophy. You can achieve your fitness and weight loss goals just by putting your mind to it!

If you've enjoyed this book, then I'd like to ask you for a favor; would you be kind enough to leave a review for this book on Amazon? It'd be greatly appreciated!

Thank you, and good luck!

Nicholas Bjorn

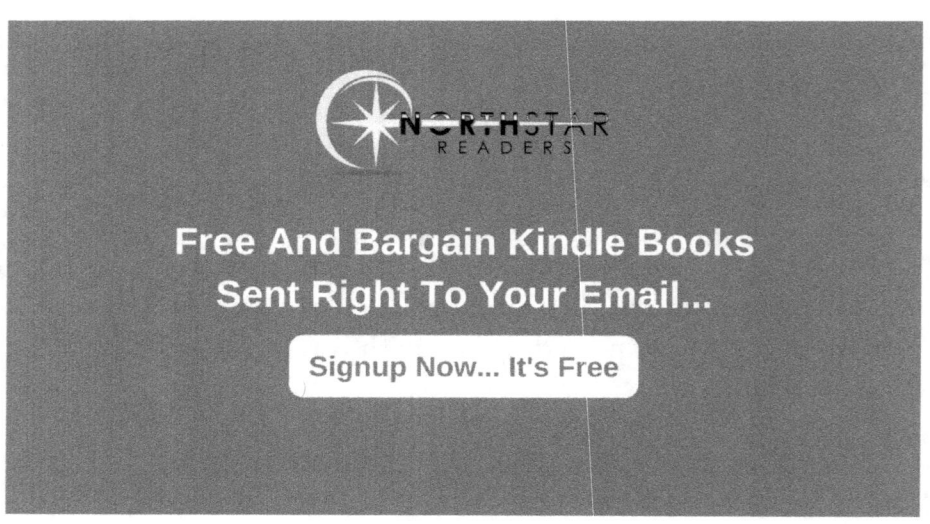

www.northstarreaders.com/reader-signup

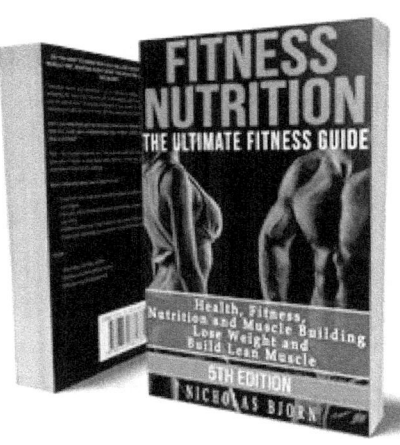

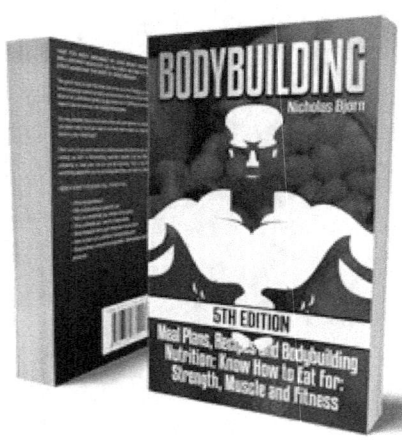

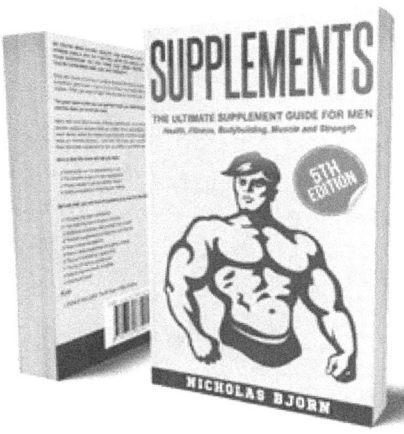